Enlightened Juicing

Meg Montañez, BCHN

Chapter 1
Juicing for Life

Meg Montañez, BCHN

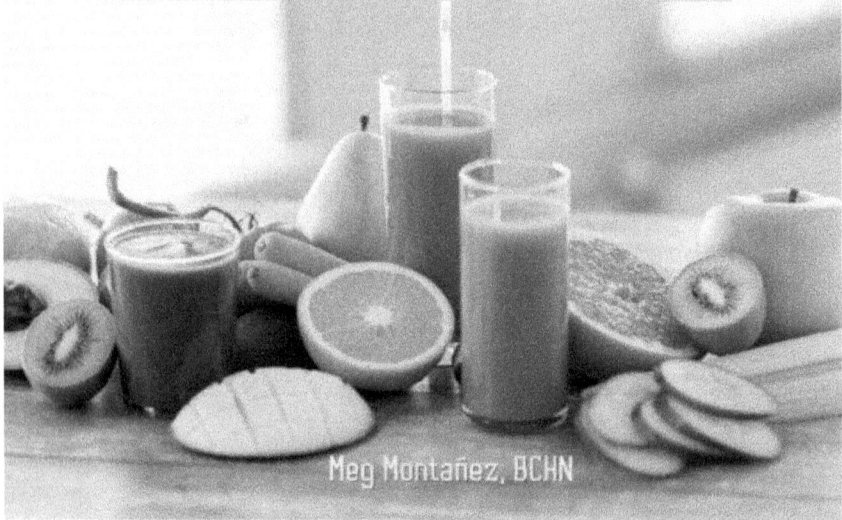

Chapter 1 – Juicing for Life

Welcome to the "Enlightened Juicing" book of seasonal recipes. Let's journey together, from season to season, through the biosphere of enlightened juicing.

The term, 'enlightened juicing', doesn't refer to any particular fruits or vegetables, juicing methods, or strategic ways of combining plant juices. Enlightened juicing has more to do with how we commune with natural foods, and especially how we can benefit most from consuming essential, plant-based nutrients in their most immaculate form; juice.

Before indulging in some tantalizing juice recipes, let's detour to your favorite imaginary grocery store, the one with the largest, and best merchandised produce section.

Every section of the store has its own energy, its own vibe. You have aisles and aisles of bottles, cans, and boxes. The food products in this part of the store are all processed. The actual food within the bottles, cans, and boxes is, at this point, dead. That is not to say that these processed food products are not packed with healthy nutrients. But processed foods have been out of the ground, or off of the tree, for far too long.

We also have the meat, fish, and poultry section. The vibe in this part of the store originates from dead animals. Enough said.

The produce section, by comparison, is different. Here, we have living plants. We have a wide array of fruits and vegetables, some of which still have their leaves and roots attached. Only a few short days ago, all of this produce was on vines, trees or in the ground. It is still, teeming with life energy. The living energy within these fruits and vegetables is a big, added plus, compared to eating processed foods. The assimilation of life energy from raw plants is one of the most significant benefits to our well-being that is associated with juicing.

Now, stand in the middle of your produce section and look around. Take a moment to regard everything. The first thing that you see is color. Lots and lots of color. We have greens, yellows, reds, blues, purples, and orange. Walk around this imaginary produce section and allow your senses to be bombarded by the aromas of these still-alive fruits and vegetables.

Color is one of the most valuable ingredients in our foods. Some may even argue that color is our foods' most valuable attribute. When we see colorful produce, we are witnessing powerful phytochemicals. These phytochemicals are classified as: flavonoids, phenolic acids, stilbenes, tannins and coumarins.

These natural colorants act as antioxidants, neutralizing molecules known as free radicals. When free radicals accumulate in the body, they create oxidative stress. They damage DNA, and can shorten a person's life.

Instead of shopping for a menu, next time you're in the grocery store, shop for color. Hmmm, this is a good day for a 'yellow fix'. Okay; bananas, yellow squash, lemons, yellow bell peppers, and corn. Oh no, let's go with a 'red fix'; apples, red bell peppers, tomatoes, red raspberries, and rhubarb…you get the idea. A 'green fix' would be a day or a meal that is loaded with chlorophyl, like spinach, green peppers, kiwi, and lettuce.

Plant Essence and Extraction

Extraction is any process that seeks to isolate and remove certain components from a particular plant. Plants have an essence, an innate life energy. Natural health experts have developed methods of extracting this energy from plant material, especially flowers. The process involves placing the flowers, or other plant material, into a bowl of pure water, then leaving the bowl in the sunlight to allow the plant essence to leach into the water. Then, the water is diluted and developed into a homeopathic remedy.

Scientists have also developed very sophisticated technologies for extracting specific biological molecules from plants, using liquid extraction mediums, such as pure water or ethanol. The process involves soaking the ground up plant material in the liquid medium for a day or two, so that the key biochemicals can leach into the medium. Then, the targeted molecules are separated from the liquid.

Being aware of this type of extraction method can be helpful when juicing fruits and vegetables, because some of the plant material can be quite dry.

Soaking jujubes, dates, or green leafy vegetables overnight, to allow for the leaching of some of the key components, is sometimes necessary, in order to create juices with a high concentration of flavorful nutrients.

Juicing is a fairly crude method of extraction, involving either the use of physical pressure, or centrifugal force. In living plants, these juices or fluids play key roles in the plant's physiology and life cycle. They transfer important biochemicals from the roots upward, and from the leaves downward. Plant fluids are a living plant's blood, marrow, and saliva. They contain concentrated components which are required for the plant's sustained life and health.

When we juice fruits and vegetables, we can see the colorful antioxidants in the juice. But there is a good bit of color remaining in the leftover plant material. This leftover plant matter still has lots of healthful nutrients. Perhaps you could make a broth with it, or maybe a neighborhood dog would like to munch on your leftover plant material. Okay then, at least mulch for your garden?

Journey into Flavors

No matter what fruits or vegetables you juice and consume, you can't go wrong. All of them have something to offer with respect to vitamins, minerals, antioxidants, and enzymes. Following the Enlightened Juicing seasonal recipe section, you will find a reference section with nutritional information about each ingredient used in the Enlightened Juicing recipes. But for the most part, the recipes themselves haven't been formulated for the purpose of achieving any specific health benefit or application. Instead, the recipes have been formulated for flavor.

Flavor is a factor in juicing we shouldn't discount. Experiencing flavors is a way we can tap into the consciousness of the plants, and plant/juice combinations. When we consume kiwi juice, for example, we're tapping into the consciousness of this rambling vine. This plump green berry is the reason for the kiwi vine's existence; it's ultimate triumph.

When juicing individual fruits and vegetables, or combinations of fruits and vegetables, the flavors can often be improved with flavor enhancers. The Enlightened Juicing recipes do not include any flavor enhancers for these reasons:

- Some enhancers are not considered to be healthy, especially for certain population groups. Therefore, adding them to natural juices and juice combinations needs to be considered in light of an individual's personal health values and dietary commitments.
- The amount and type of enhancer desired is a matter of personal taste.

With respect to juices, flavor enhancers are mainly used for two reasons:

1. to add extra sweetness to a tart or sour fruit

2.   to mask the bitterness of certain vegetables and vegetable combinations

Bitterness:

Some juice enthusiasts combine fruits in with their vegetable juices, like apple or pear. They add some sweet flavor as a way to mask bitterness. In the Enlightened Juicing recipes, we have only rarely mixed fruits in with vegetables. Experiencing vegetables in their natural state is the best way to tune into the consciousness of the vegetable. Embrace a little bitterness. However, there are ways to mask bitterness with herbs, such as:

- ginger

- mint

- basil

- coriander

- curry (try this!)

Another consideration is salt. Some people should not consume salt, or only use it in small quantities. If you want to add some salt, use sea salt. You could also experiment with soy sauce or tamari.

Sweetness:

Fruits contain natural sugars, but some contain more than others. Juice enthusiasts often choose to add a little sweetener to fruit juices. These include:

- Sugar, in all of its forms, including processed white and raw sugar, is an effective sweetener, but is considered taboo by many nutritionists. It is especially risky for anyone suffering from any form of blood glucose imbalance. If you use sugar, use it sparingly. Use cane sugar, and do not use fructose.

- Stevia is a super-sweet biochemical which is extracted from the plant, Stevia rebaudiana. It is not a sugar and is considered a benign, zero calorie sweetener, occurring naturally in the leaves of this shrub. The consumption of small amounts of stevia is generally considered as safe by the FDA.

- Maple syrup is a healthy alternative to sugar, but it adds a distinctive flavor to your juice, which may or may not be desirable.

- Molasses is a form of unprocessed sugar that can be a good alternative to processed sugar. It too, however, has its own distinctive flavor.

If your juices come out a little thick, like persimmon juice for example, you can always add an ounce of pure water.

Juicing and Fasting

Fasting is an essential component to a healthy metabolism. Fasting begins when all recently consumed food has been completely digested. The body needs this fasting time to process and utilize glycogen and fats. Our bodies have evolved to require periods of fasting in order to maintain our metabolic health.

Consuming juices alone, without solid food, is considered by many fasting counselors as a form of fasting. When we consume only juices, our digestive system is only moderately engaged, leaving the body with plenty of energy for other purposes. Juices assimilate quickly, allowing the fasting period to remain engaged. Juices are the purest, most highly concentrated form of nutritious food that we have available to us.

Seasonal Recipes

The Enlightened Juicing collection is organized by season of the year. Each recipe uses fruits and vegetables that are normally harvested and consumed in a particular season. Fruits and vegetables that are defined by a particular season, like kiwi, cranberry, melons, and persimmon, are featured within their harvest season, both as a singular ingredient, and in combination with other compatible fruits. This will allow you to enjoy a particular fruit or vegetable that you especially like, either by itself, or with a variety of partners, and then decide which combination you prefer.

Within each recipe, that combines two or more juices, each juice plays a distinct role. Sweet fruits are combined with sour and tart fruits, to keep the sweetness factor elevated. Fr example, some juices, like watermelon, grape, apple, and pear are used as sweet bases for other more flavorful juices, such as berries, persimmons, kiwi, and pomegranates.

Enjoy!

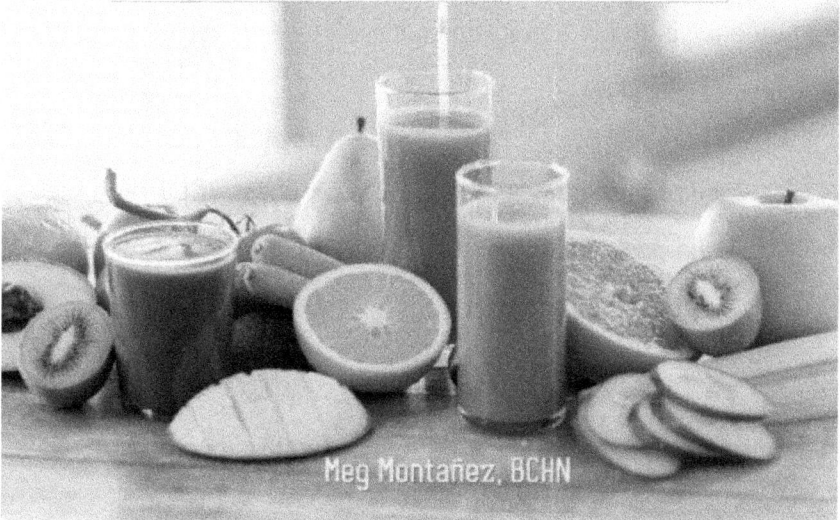

Enlightened Juicing
Chapter 2
The Fall Recipes

Meg Montañez, BCHN

Chapter 2 – The Fall Recipes

Fall #1 – Date / Strawberry / Raspberry

Try this tasty berry-ade, in a base of sugary date water.

Preparation:

- soak eight pitted dates overnight in 6 ounces of purified water

- slice ½ pint of strawberries

- 3 ounces of raspberries

Juice:

- juice eight dates, along with the date water, together with the berries

Fall #2 – Date / Lemon / Lime

There's a reason why soft drink bottlers combine lemon and lime. It works. Now, add those two tart citrus favorites with the sugary date, and you have a divine lemon/limeade.

Preparation:

- soak eight pitted dates overnight in 6 ounces of purified water

- slice and peel one lemon and cut into quarters

- slice and peel one lime and cut into quarters

Juice:

- juice eight dates, along with the date water, together with a peeled ¼ lemon wedge and a peeled ¼ lime wedge

Fall #3 – Apple / Pear / Persimmon

When apple and pear are mixed together, they produce a unique-tasting, sweet blend that acts as an excellent base for distinctive flavors, like persimmon. This recipe will yield about 10-12 ounces of juice, and can be cut in half, if desirable.

Preparation:

- slice three ripe persimmons, unpeeled

- slice two unpeeled apples

- slice two unpeeled pears

Juice:

- juice the apple and pear slices, together with the persimmon wedges

Fall #4 – Date / Pomegranate

The pomegranate is another tart/sweet fruit that thrives in combination with the sweet date. Preparing a pomegranate for juicing is time-consuming, yet worth the effort.

Preparation:

- soak eight pitted dates overnight in 6 ounces of purified water
- without cutting too deeply, cut a circle around the top of the outer pomegranate rind of one fruit, and lift the top off
- cut a second circle around the pomegranate bottom and remove it
- make shallow slices in the side of the pomegranate, along the lines of the white inner pith
- break the pomegranate apart into three or more sections
- carefully remove the outer rind, and the white inner pith

Juice:

- juice the eight dates along with the date water, together with the pomegranate seeds collected, still surrounded by their outer membranes (arils)

Fall #5 - Jujube / Ginger / Cinnamon

While the jujube, or 'red date', is sweet, it contains only about half of the sugar of a date, and has an earthier flavor. A little seasoning is all the jujube needs.

Preparation:

   - soak ten pitted jujubes overnight in six ounces of purified water

Juice:

   - juice the ten jujubes along with the jujube water, with an added dash of ginger and an added dash of cinnamon

Fall #6 – Apple / Pear / Strawberry

When apple and pear are mixed together, they produce a unique-tasting, sweet blend that acts as an excellent base for distinctive flavors, like strawberry. This recipe will yield about 10-12 ounces of juice, and can be cut in half, if desirable.

Preparation:

   - slice two unpeeled apples
   - slice two unpeeled pears
   - slice ½ pint of raw, ripe strawberries

Juice:

   - juice apples, pears, and strawberries together

Fall #7 – Apple / Pear / Pomegranate

When apple and pear are mixed together, they produce a unique-tasting, sweet blend that acts as an excellent base for distinctive flavors, like pomegranate. This recipe will yield about 10 ounces of juice.

Preparation:

- without cutting too deeply, cut a circle around the top of the outer pomegranate rind of one fruit, and lift the top off

- cut a second circle around the pomegranate bottom and remove

- make shallow slices in the sides of the pomegranate, along the lines of the white inner pith

- break the pomegranate apart into three or more sections

- carefully remove the outer rind and the white pith

- slice two unpeeled apples and two unpeeled pears

Juice:

- juice the apple and pear slices, together with the pomegranate seeds collected, still surrounded by their outer membranes (arils)

Fall #8 – Date / Kiwi

The complex tart/sweet kiwi thrives in the date's sugary base.

Preparation:

- soak eight pitted dates overnight in 6 ounces of purified water

- slice three ripe kiwis, without peeling

Juice:

- juice eight dates, along with the date water, together with the kiwis

---

Fall #9 – Dark or Concord Grape / Pomegranate

The slightly tart pomegranate's flavor comes to life in a base of fresh, sweet grape juice.

Preparation:

- wash 30 colorful grapes
- without cutting too deeply, cut a circle around the top of the outer pomegranate rind of one fruit, and lift the top off
- repeat cutting a second circle around the pomegranate bottom and remove the bottom
- make shallow slices in the sides of the pomegranate, along the lines of the white inner pith
- break the pomegranate apart into three or more sections
- carefully remove the outer rind
- carefully remove as much of the white pith as possible

Juice:

- juice the grapes, together with the pomegranate seeds collected, still surrounded by their outer membranes (arils)

Fall #10 – Dark or Concord Grape / Blackberries

Blackberries lack a bit in sweetness, compared to their cousins, like raspberries and boysenberries, but combining them with sweet grape juice makes their distinctive flavor shine.

Preparation:

- wash 30 colorful grapes
- wash 3 ounces of blackberries

Juice:

- juice the berries together with the grapes

Fall #11 – Mandarin Orange / Lime

The Mandarin is one of nature's sweetest citrus fruits. Adding some sour lime makes the Mandarin come alive.

Preparation:

- peel eight Mandarin oranges and separate sections
- peel a lime and slice into quarters.

Juice:

- juice one quarter lime with eight Mandarin oranges

Fall #12 – Watermelon / Pomegranate

Another great match-up for the pomegranate is the neutral watermelon base.

Preparation:

- remove the rind from one and one-half pounds of watermelon
- without cutting too deeply, cut a circle around the top of the outer pomegranate rind of one fruit, and lift the top off
- repeat cutting a second circle around the pomegranate bottom and remove the bottom
- make shallow slices in the sides of the pomegranate, along the lines of the white inner pith
- break the pomegranate apart into three or more sections
- carefully remove the outer rind
- carefully remove as much of the white pith as possible

Juice:

- juice the watermelon, together with the pomegranate seeds collected, still surrounded by their outer membranes (arils)

Fall #13 – Watermelon / Persimmon

The sweet persimmon, with the mild watermelon, are a perfect match.

Preparation:

- remove the rind from one and one-half pounds of watermelon
- slice three ripe persimmons, unpeeled

Juice:

- juice the watermelon, together with the sliced persimmons

Fall #14 – Peach / Nectarine / Pomegranate

The peach and nectarine provide, yet another delicious, sweet blended base for the tangy pomegranate.

Preparation:

- slice one unpeeled, ripe nectarine
- slice one unpeeled, ripe peach
- without cutting too deeply, cut a circle around the top of the outer pomegranate rind of one fruit, and lift the top off
- cut a second circle around the pomegranate bottom and remove
- make shallow slices in the sides of the pomegranate, along the lines of the white inner pith
- break the pomegranate apart into three or more sections
- carefully remove the outer rind
- carefully remove as much of the white pith as possible

Juice:

- juice the peach and nectarine, together with the collected pomegranate seeds, still surrounded by their outer membranes (arils)

Fall #15 - Tomato / Squash / Celery / Radish

In this blend, the squash (your favorite type) gives character to the tomato and celery, with radish providing the kick.

Preparation:

- slice an average-sized ripe tomato

- wash four celery stalks

- slice one average-sized zucchini, or similar squash

- slice one average-sized radish

Juice:

- juice all four vegetable ingredients together

Fall #16 - Celery / Burdock Root / Cilantro / Ginger

Burdock, cilantro, and ginger make an exquisite flavor blend, in a base of mild celery juice.

Preparation:

- clean and slice a 1" slice of ginger root

- clean and slice six inches of burdock root

- clean and prepare five celery stalks

- clean and prepare eight cilantro stems/leaves

Juice:

- juice the celery first, then the ginger, then burdock, then cilantro

Fall #17 - Celery / Leek / Bell Pepper

Leek adds tangy flavor to the bell pepper, in a base of mild celery.

Preparation:

- clean and slice a medium-sized leek

- clean and slice a bell pepper, your choice of color

- clean and prepare five celery stalks

Juice:

- juice the celery first, then the leek with leaves, and the pepper

Fall #18 - Cucumber / Rhubarb / Tomato / Green Onion / Chile Pepper

The mild cucumber and tomato are enhanced with green onion and chile pepper. Follow preparation instructions, using only about one sixth of an average-sized jalapeno pepper.

Preparation:

- clean and slice one average-sized cucumber

- clean and prepare four stalks of rhubarb

- clean and slice one tomato

- clean and prepare six green onions

- slice off a small piece of chile pepper, about one sixth of a pepper

Juice:

- juice the tomato, then the cucumber, then rhubarb, onion, and pepper

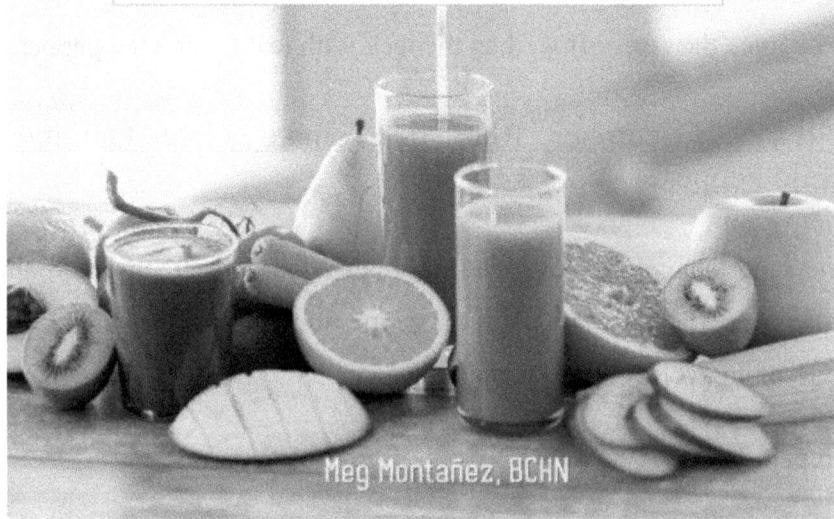

Enlightened Juicing
Chapter 3
The Winter Recipes

Meg Montañez, BCHN

Chapter 3 – The Winter Recipes

Winter #1 – Kiwi

"Make mine straight kiwi". Discover the unique, magical taste of this plump, green, Asian berry, grown on a rambling vine. Start with three kiwis, and then if you hear the bells go off, next time, juice four.

Preparation:

- wash and slice three ripe, unpeeled kiwis

Juice:

- run the kiwis through the juicer and enjoy

Winter #2 – Orange / Kiwi

With Kiwi's distinct taste, containing only a modest amount of sugar, adding a sweeter juice as a partner, like orange, only enhances kiwi's allure. Mandarin oranges and blood oranges could be substituted.

Preparation:

- wash and slice two ripe, unpeeled kiwis
- peel two juice oranges and slice

Juice:

- put the oranges through the juicer first, followed by the kiwis

Winter #3 – Grapefruit / Kiwi

Pairing kiwi with grapefruit is another variation on the same citrus/kiwi theme, with the grapefruit acting as a sweeter base. If this combination receives high marks, the recipe can be doubled the second time around.

Preparation:

- peel and slice one large grapefruit, white or red
- wash and slice one ripe, unpeeled kiwi

Juice:

- put the grapefruit through the juicer first, followed by the kiwi.

Winter #4 – Grape / Kiwi

Another sweet base for kiwi is grape juice. Use either green table grapes or darker grapes. Kiwis and grapes make a great team.

Preparation:

- clean thirty grapes
- clean and slice two ripe, unpeeled kiwis

Juice:

- put the grapes through the juicer, followed by the kiwis

Winter #5 – Lemon / Lime / Dark Grape / Kiwi

This combination is a variation on Winter #4, with lemon and lime added, for extra zest.

Preparation:

- clean thirty dark grapes
- clean and slice two ripe, unpeeled kiwis
- peel and quarter one lemon
- peel and quarter one lime

Juice:

- juice grapes, followed by two kiwis
- juice a one-quarter lime wedge

- juice a one-quarter lemon wedge

Winter #6 – Persimmon

Discover the decadent pleasure of straight persimmon juice. The gods will be jealous.

Preparation:

- remove leaves from two ripe persimmons, without removing skin

Juice:

- slice and juice both fruits

Winter #7 – Lemon / Persimmon

Persimmons are sweet enough on their own, so that you can add some lemon and experiment with persimmon lemonade.

Preparation:

- remove leaves from two ripe, unpeeled persimmons
- peel and quarter one lemon

Juice:

- slice and juice the persimmons
- juice a one quarter lemon wedge

Winter #8 – Grape / Persimmon

Grape's added sugar combines with persimmon for a sweet treat.

Preparation:

- clean thirty grapes, white or dark
- remove leaves from one ripe, unpeeled persimmon and slice

Juice:

- juice grapes first, then add sliced persimmon

Winter #9 – Pomelo

Pomelos are often confused with grapefruits. Discover the uniquely sweet flavor of the pomelo.

Preparation:

- peel one pomelo and break into sections

Juice:

- juice one fruit, but have a second on stand-by

Winter #10 – Pomelo / Kiwi

The pomelo provides a uniquely sweet, slightly tart base for the exotic kiwi.

Preparation:

- peel one pomelo and break into sections
- clean and slice one ripe, unpeeled kiwi

Juice:

- juice the pomelo first, followed by the kiwi

Winter #11 – Mandarin Orange

Discover the mandarin all by itself, the orange family's sweetest, most flavorful cousin.

Preparation:

- peel five Mandarin oranges and separate into sections

Juice:

- juice and enjoy

Winter #12 – Mandarin Orange / Persimmon

The Mandarin's sweetness creates a great base for the dreamy persimmon.

Preparation:

- peel three Mandarin oranges and separate into sections
- remove leaves from two ripe, unpeeled persimmons and slice

Juice:

- juice the mandarins first
- juice the persimmons

Winter #13 – Grape / Cranberry / Lemon

Cranberries are a healthy, flavorful, yet tart fruit. Juicing them at home is unpractical for most people, since the process is multi-phased, and requires cooking the cranberries. For this recipe, it is recommended to purchase raw, unsweetened cranberry juice. Grape provides a sweet base, and the lemon gives the combination a lemony flair.

Preparation:

- wash twenty-five dark or green grapes

- peel and quarter one lemon

- prepare two ounces of raw cranberry juice

Juice:

- juice the grapes

- juice the lemon wedge

- mix in the two ounces of cranberry juice

Winter #14 – Blood Orange – Persimmon – Red Grape – Red Pomelo (*red fix*)

Two of these red fruits, blood oranges and red pomelos, are both slightly sour. Combined with sweet grape and persimmon, it results in a unique, seductive flavor.

Preparation:

- peel and section one blood orange

- remove leaves from one ripe, unpeeled persimmon and slice

- clean ten red grapes

- peel a red pomelo and break into sections

Juice:

- juice the red pomelo and blood orange first

- juice the red grapes

- add persimmon slices to juicer

Winter #15 – Mandarin Orange / Cranberry

Cranberries are a healthy, flavorful, yet tart fruit. Juicing them at home is unpractical for most people, since the process is multi-phased, and requires cooking the cranberries. For this recipe, it is recommended to purchase raw, unsweetened cranberry juice. Mandarin oranges provide a sweet base for the cranberries, but other varieties of orange could be substituted, including blood oranges.

Preparation:

- peel and section four Mandarin oranges

- measure two ounces of cranberry juice

Juice:

- juice the Mandarins

- mix in two ounces of cranberry juice

Winter #16 – Carrot / Spinach / Green Onion / Green Lettuce / Fennel / Endive

Enjoy this tasty, slightly bitter, green-dominant liquid salad, packed with healthy nutrients.

Preparation:

- wash eight medium-sized carrots
- wash and prepare three green onions
- wash and break apart three lettuce leaves
- wash and break apart eight spinach leaves
- wash and break apart three endive leaves
- wash and slice one fennel stalk

Juice:

- juice the carrots first
- juice the entire green onions, including roots
- juice the green leaves

Winter #17 – Carrot / Broccoli / Squash / Radish

This unique liquid salad combination benefits from the warm, spicy radish, with minimal bitterness.

Preparation:

- wash eight medium-sized carrots
- wash and break apart one half of a broccoli head

- wash and slice a medium-sized squash (zucchini, summer squash)

- clean and section one radish

Winter #18 – Carrot / Beet / Radish / Green Onion / Sprout Grass

The sweet carrot base helps offset the earthy beet and the bitter sprout and onion grass, while the radish adds zest.

Preparation:

- wash eight medium-sized carrots

- wash and slice one medium-sized beet, with skins intact

- wash and section one radish

- wash three green onions

- wash one ounce of sprout grass with roots (wheat, barley, alfalfa)

Juice:

- begin juicing the carrots, followed by the beet

- juice the radish

- juice the three onions

- juice the sprout grass last

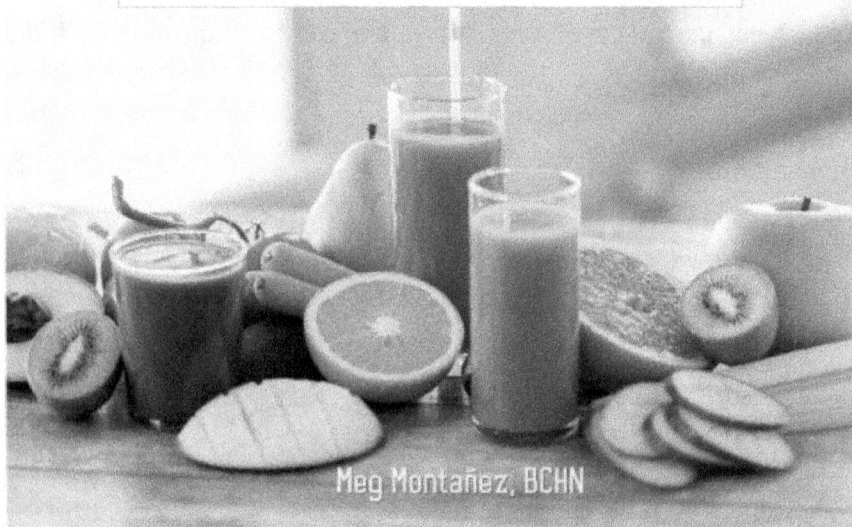

Enlightened Juicing
Chapter 4
The Spring Recipes

Meg Montañez, BCHN

Chapter 4 – The Spring Recipes

Spring #1 – Peach

Fresh peach juice is another exotic taste treat that many never experience. Start with two peaches, and if the bells go off, juice three next time.

Preparation:

  - wash, pit and slice two ripe peaches

Juice:

- juice the peach slices

Spring #2 – Nectarine

Like fresh peach juice, fresh nectarine juice is another exotic pleasure that few have taken the time to experience. And no, it's not the same as peach juice.

Preparation:

- wash, pit and slice two ripe nectarines

Juice:

- juice the nectarine slices

Spring #3 – Peach / Plum

Peach and plum make tasty partners.

Preparation:

- wash and slice one ripe peach
- wash and slice four ripe plums

Juice:

- juice the plums
- juice the peaches

Spring #4 – Cherry

Raw cherry juice requires an extra step, in order to remove the cherry pits.

Preparation:

- place two cups of cherries into a mixing bowl and smash with spoon
- add ½ ounce of pure water and mix with cherries
- place the cherry mash into blender and set blender to low
- blend the cherry mash until the pits are all separated from the fruit, but the pits are still intact
- remove pits with fork or strainer

Juice:

- put the pitted mash through the juicer

Spring #5 – Pomelo / Cherry

Raw cherry juice is a true delicacy, but requires an extra step, in order to remove the cherry pits.

Preparation:

- follow the directions in Spring #4 for creating a cherry mash with two cups of cherries
- peel and section one pomelo

Juice:

- juice the pitted cherry mash first, followed by the pomelo

Spring #6 – Pomelo / Strawberry / Raspberry

The strawberry and raspberry add a wonderful flavor to the sweet pomelo. You could use both berries for their combined flavor, or you could use only one. If you choose to use only one, double the berry content to six ounces of raspberries or ten ripe strawberries.

Preparation:

- peel and section one pomelo
- prepare three ounces of raspberries
- wash and slice six ripe strawberries

Juice:

- juice the pomelo
- juice the strawberries
- juice the raspberries

Spring #7 – Pomelo / Blueberry / Blackberry

The blueberry and blackberry add a wonderful flavor to the sweet pomelo. You could use both berries for their combined flavor, or you could use only one. If you choose to use only one, double the berry content to six ounces of blueberries or six ounces of blackberries.

Preparation:

- peel and section one pomelo
- prepare three ounces of blueberries

- prepare three ounces of blackberries

Juice:

- juice the pomelo
- juice the berries

Spring #8 – Pomelo / Lemon / Lime / Strawberry

This combination produces a strawberry lemon/limeade, with a sweet pomelo base.

Preparation:

- peel and section one pomelo
- wash and slice eight ripe strawberries
- peel and quarter one lemon
- peel and quarter one lime

Juice:

- juice the pomelo sections
- juice the lemon and lime wedges
- juice the strawberries

Spring #9 – Nectarine / Cherry / Lemon

Nectarine is a flavorful, sweet base for cherry lemonade. As an alternative to processing your own cherry juice, raw, unsweetened cherry juice can also be obtained in bottled form.

Preparation:

- place one cup of cherries into a mixing bowl and smash with a big spoon

- add ¼ ounce of pure water and mix with cherries

- place the cherry mash into blender and run blender on low

- blend the cherry mash until the pits are all separated from the fruit, but the pits are still intact

- remove pits with fork or strainer

- wash, pit and slice one ripe nectarine

- peel and quarter one lemon

Juice:

- juice the cherry mash first

- juice the lemon wedge

- juice the nectarine last

Spring #10 – Nectarine / Apricot

The sweeter nectarine provides an ideal base for the drier and flavorful apricot.

Preparation:

- wash, pit and slice one ripe nectarine

- wash, pit and slice five ripe apricots

Juice:

- juice the apricots first

- juice the nectarine

Spring #11 – Red Grapefruit / Strawberry / Rhubarb / Cherry / Red Raspberry / Cranberry (*red fix*)

This red fix combination uses six red fruits. However, you may only have four or five of these fruits available. This recipe assumes you will probably use only four or five of these ingredients. Bear in mind, if you use all six, it will result in a tall glass of juice. Perhaps you can split it with someone? Raw cranberry juice will probably have to be obtained in bottled form. Raw cherry juice is also available in bottled form.

Preparation:

- peel and section one half red grapefruit
- wash and slice four ripe strawberries
- wash and prepare two rhubarb stalks
- prepare three ounces of raspberries
- wash, pit, and mash eight cherries

Juice:

- juice strawberries first
- juice rhubarb stalks
- juice raspberries
- juice cherries
- juice grapefruit last
- mix in two ounces of raw cranberry juice

Spring #12 – Orange / Strawberry

The flavorful strawberry combines well with the sweet and juicy orange. In addition to good juice oranges, experiment with Mandarin orange and blood oranges.

Preparation:

- peel and section two large, or three medium-sized oranges

- wash and slice ten average-sized, ripe strawberries

Juice:

- juice the strawberries first, followed by the orange wedges

Spring #13 – Celery / Carrot / Chile Pepper / Radish

With radish and a bit of chile pepper, this celery/carrot combo is a spice lover's delight. Do not; repeat, do not juice an entire jalapeno pepper.

Preparation:

- separate and wash four celery stalks

- wash five average-sized carrots

- wash and slice one radish

- slice one-sixth of an average-sized jalapeno pepper, or comparable variety of chile pepper

Juice:

- juice the carrots first

- juice the radish

- juice the slice of chile pepper (one-sixth of the entire pepper)

- juice the celery stalks

Spring #14 – Celery / Broccoli / Dandelion Green / Green Onion / Green Lettuce / Collard Green / Spinach / Kale / Sprout Grass (*green fix*)

This recipe is a green fix, with lots of nutrients, plenty of chlorophyl, and the expected bitterness. You may want to consider masking the bitterness with some potent flavors, such as salt, ginger, or fennel.

Preparation:

- wash four celery stalks

- wash and slice one half broccoli head

- wash three green onions

- prepare the following green leaves by chopping them and soaking them overnight in three ounces of water:

  o six dandelion leaves

  o four green lettuce leaves

  o three collard green leaves

  o six spinach leaves

  o three kale leaves

  o ¼ ounce sprout grass (wheat, barley, alfalfa)

Juice:

- juice the broccoli head

- juice the green onions

- juice the chopped leaves' mash, with mash water

- juice the four celery stalks

Spring #15 – Celery / Cilantro / Green Onion

This simple combination has a cilantro-dominant flavor, enhanced by the onion.

Preparation:

- wash five celery stalks

- wash four green onions

- wash 1/4 to 1/3 of a typical grocery store bunch of cilantro

Juice:

- juice the onions

- juice the cilantro

- juice the celery stalks

Spring #16 – Carrot / Tomato / Leek / Radish / Turnip

Another great liquid salad combination, the leek, radish, and turnip provide a tasty character to the carrot and tomato base.

Preparation:

- wash five average-sized carrots

- wash and slice one average-sized tomato

- wash two leek stalks

- wash and slice one radish

- wash and slice one turnip

Juice:

- juice the carrots first

- juice the leek stalks

- juice the radish

- juice the turnip

- juice the tomato slices

Spring #17 – Celery / Cauliflower / Chard / Leek

Chard and leek provide a combination similar to green onion and garlic, except that they are both sweeter and less bitter. The cauliflower combines with the celery for a unique-tasting, somewhat neutral base.

Preparation:

- wash, separate, and chop 1/3 head of cauliflower

- wash and separate four celery stalks

- wash and chop five chard leaves/stalks

- wash two leek stalks

Juice:

- juice the leek stalks

- juice the five chard leaves

- juice the cauliflower

- juice the celery stalks

Spring #18 – Celery / Shallot / Tomato / Garlic / Lemon

With shallot and garlic, this celery/tomato combination is full of flavor.

Preparation:

- wash and slice one average-sized tomato (1/2 pound)
- wash three celery stalks
- wash and chop one shallot
- separate and peel two cloves of garlic
- peel and quarter one lemon

Juice:

- juice the tomato first
- juice the shallot and the garlic cloves
- juice the celery stalks
- juice the lemon wedge

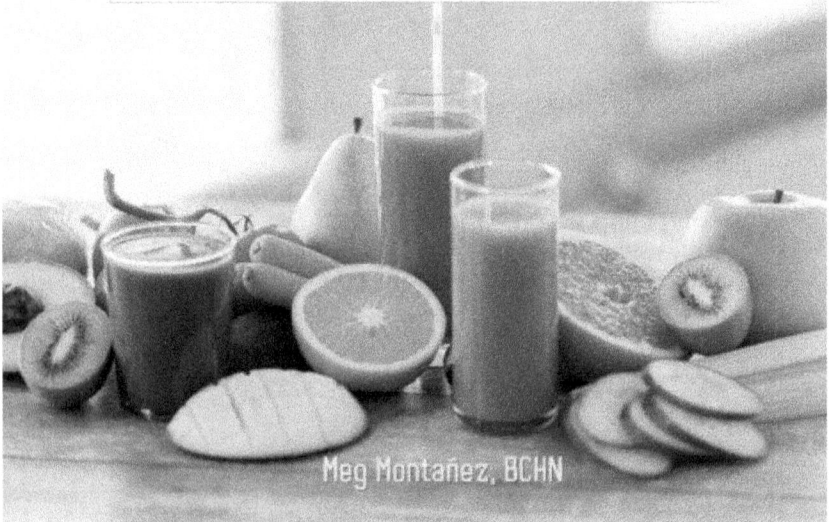

Enlightened Juicing
Chapter 5
The Summer Recipes

Chapter 5 – The Summer Recipes

Summer #1 – Watermelon / Casaba Melon / Honeydew Melon

Okay, here's your chance to channel your inner melon. These three combined create a delightful flavorful blend. This recipe will yield a tall glass of juice.

Preparation:

- peel and slice one eighth of an average-sized watermelon
- peel and slice one fourth of an average-sized casaba melon

- peel and slice one fourth of an average-sized honeydew melon

Juice:

- juice the honeydew, the casaba, and then the watermelon

Summer #2 – Watermelon – Blueberry – Raspberry – Strawberry

The juicy watermelon provides a neutral base for the sweet, tart berries. Use a total of six ounces of berries. If you use all three, two ounces each. If one, use six ounces. The recipe below will yield a tall glass of juice.

Preparation:

- peel and slice one-sixth of an average-sized watermelon
- wash and slice two ounces of strawberries
- wash two ounces of blueberries
- prepare two ounces of raspberries

Summer #3 – Watermelon / Strawberry / Cherry / Red Grape / Rhubarb (*red fix*)

This blend is a summertime red fix, using the watery watermelon as a neutral base.

Preparation:

- peel and slice one eighth of an average-sized watermelon
- wash and slice six average-sized ripe strawberries

- wash ten red grapes

- wash two rhubarb stalks

- wash and prepare ten cherries according to the instructions in Winter recipe #1, or prepare two ounces of raw cherry juice

Juice:

- juice grapes

- juice rhubarb

- juice strawberries

- juice watermelon

- juice cherry mash, or add two ounces of raw cherry juice (bottled)

Summer #4 – Apple / Blueberry / Boysenberry / Raspberry

Apples are never better than when they're combined with berries in a cool summer refresher. This recipe will yield a tall glass of juice.

Preparation:

- wash and slice two sweet apples

- wash three ounces of blueberries

- wash three ounces of boysenberries

- wash three ounces of raspberries

Summer #5 – Black or Concord Grape / Plum / Blackberry / Boysenberry (*purple fix*)

This blend is a summertime purple fix.

Preparation:

- wash twenty black or concord grapes

- wash, pit, and slice three ripe plums

- prepare three ounces of blackberries

- prepare three ounces of boysenberries

Juice:

- juice the plums first

- juice the berries

- juice the grapes last

Summer #6 – Apple / Cherry / Lime

A great sweet and sour summer treat. The choice of apples should be focused on sweeter varieties, such as red delicious or Fuji.

Preparation:

- wash and slice two apples

- peel and quarter one lime

- prepare cherry mash with ten cherries, according to instructions in Winter recipe #1, or prepare two ounces of raw cherry juice (bottled)

Juice:

- juice the lime

- juice the apple slices

- juice the cherry mash, or mix in two ounces of bottled cherry juice

Summer #7 – Pear / Apricot

The ripe, summer pear provides a sweet backdrop for the flavorful apricot.

Preparation:

- wash and slice two ripe pears
- wash and slice eight ripe apricots

Juice:

- juice the apricots, then juice the pears

Summer #8 – Pear / Nectarine

The ripe, summer pear provides an excellent base for the sweet, flavorful nectarine.

Preparation:

- wash and slice two ripe pears
- wash and slice two ripe nectarines

Juice:

- juice the nectarines first, then juice the pears

Summer #9 – Pear / Peach / Boysenberry / Blackberry / Blueberry

The ripe, summer pear provides an excellent base for the sweet, juicy peach. Add the berries for a big splash of flavor. Use one or all of the berry varieties, with the total berry weight approximately six ounces, combined. The recipe here assumes the inclusion of all three berry varieties.

Preparation:

- wash and slice one ripe pear

- wash and slice two ripe peaches

- wash and prepare a total of six ounces of berries, using boysenberry, blackberry, and/or blueberry

Summer #10 – Pear / Plum

The sweet pear base allows for the expressive taste of the plum to shine.

Preparation:

- wash and slice one ripe pear

- wash and slice four ripe plums

Juice:

- juice the plums, followed by the pear

Summer #11 – Peach / Nectarine / Plum / Apricot

Nothing says summertime better than this four-stone-fruit combination. The apricot benefits from its sweeter relatives. The recipe below will yield a tall glass of juice.

Preparation:

- wash, pit and slice one ripe peach
- wash, pit and slice one ripe nectarine
- wash, pit and slice two ripe plums
- wash, pit and slice four ripe apricots

Juice:

- juice the peach, the nectarine, and the apricots first
- juice the plums last

Summer #12 – Pear / Strawberry / Lemon

Strawberry lemonade, with pear as a sweet base.

Preparation:

- wash and slice two ripe pears
- wash and slice eight medium-sized strawberries
- peel and quarter one lemon

Juice:

- juice the strawberries first

- juice two of the lemon quarter wedges

- juice the two pears last

Summer #13 – Black or Concord Grape / Lemon / Lime

Another summer treat; grape lemon-limeade.

Preparation:

- wash forty black or concord grapes

- peel and quarter one lemon

- peel and quarter one lime

Juice:

- juice one lemon quarter

- juice one lime quarter

- juice forty grapes

Summer #14 – Black or Concord Grape / Nectarine / Plum

Grape provides a sweet base for two of the sweetest stone fruits, nectarine and plum. No extra sugar needed here. This recipe will yield a tall glass of juice.

Preparation:

- wash twenty concord or black grapes

- wash and slice one ripe nectarine

- wash and slice two ripe plums

Juice:

- juice the grapes first

- juice the nectarine

- juice the two plums

Summer #15 – Concord Grape

If you think you've experienced concord grape juice, having only consumed it processed and bottled; no. If you haven't enjoyed homemade, natural concord grape juice, you haven't experienced it at all.

Preparation:

- wash forty concord grapes

Juice:

- juice the grapes

Summer #16 / Carrot / Tomato / Green Chile Pepper / Radish / Leek

This summer salad is packed with flavor; spicy! Do not; repeat, do not juice an entire chile pepper.

Preparation:

- slice one-sixth of an average-sized jalapeno pepper, or comparable variety of chile pepper

- wash and slice one radish

- wash one leek stalk

- wash and slice one average-sized tomato

- wash and prepare six average-sized carrots

Summer #17 – Celery / Cucumber / Green Lettuce / Green Bell Pepper (*green fix*)

This liquid summer salad is another green fix, but one low on the bitterness scale.

Preparation:

- wash five celery stalks
- wash and slice one bell pepper
- wash and slice one cucumber (unpeeled)
- wash and chop six green lettuce leaves

Juice:

- juice the bell pepper
- juice the cucumber
- juice the chopped lettuce leaves
- juice the celery stalks

Summer #18 – Celery / Green Bell Pepper / Tomatillos / Green Onion / Spinach (*green fix*)

This summer salad is a green fix, with all ingredients providing chlorophyl. The bitter green may need to be offset somewhat with a strong flavor additive, such as fennel, ginger, or mint.

Preparation:

- wash eight spinach leaves and chop

- add two ounces of pure water to chopped spinach and let sit overnight

- wash four celery stalks

- wash and slice one green bell pepper

- wash and slice one tomatillo

- wash and prepare three green onions

Juice:

- juice tomatillo

- juice green onions

- juice bell pepper

- juice spinach leaf mash

- juice four celery stalks

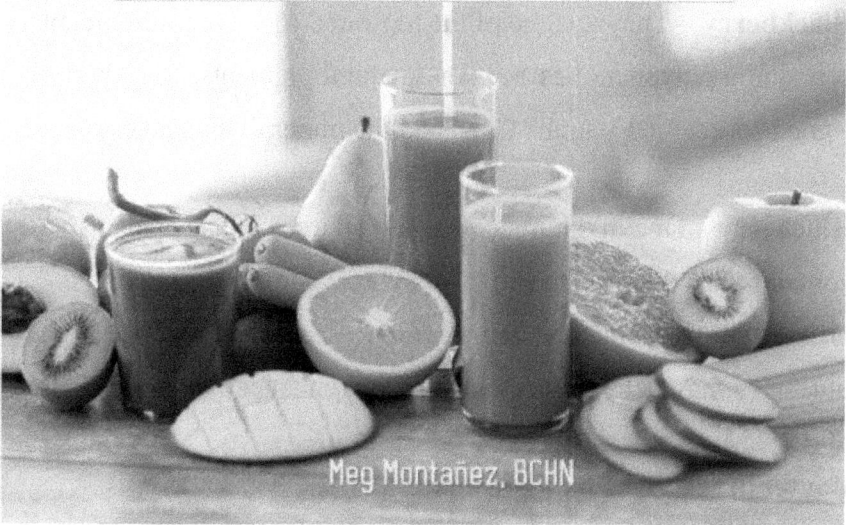

Enlightened Juicing

Chapter 6
Nutritional Compendium

Meg Montañez, BCHN

Chapter 6 – Nutritional Compendium

Here's a quick reference list of Enlightened Juicing ingredients, in alphabetical order, with some enlightening nutritional facts and information.

Fruits:

Apple – Along with being a good source for vitamin C, apples contain pectin, which aids digestion, and the antioxidant, quercetin.

Apricot – An excellent source of Vitamins A and C, plus the minerals, potassium, magnesium and iron. They're also an excellent source the antioxidants carotene, lycopene, and lutein. Researchers believe that apricots are great for enhancing vision and may have anti-cancer effects.

Blackberry – They are one of the top-rated foods for antioxidants, containing polyphenolics and other natural pigments. Blackberry is a good source of Vitamins C, K, and the mineral, manganese.

Blueberry – One of nature's very best sources of antioxidants, containing as many as twenty-five anthocyanins, which also provide anti-inflammatory protection. Researchers believe that the blueberry may help protect the brain and enhance longevity.

Boysenberry – The nutritional profile of the boysenberry is similar to the blackberry.

Casaba Melon – Very high in Vitamin C, B6, thiamin, niacin, and folate, casaba is also packed with the minerals, potassium and copper, thought to be good for great-looking skin.

Cherry – Along with being a good source of Vitamin C, cherries are packed with nutritious phytochemicals, including quercetin and anthocyanidins. Researchers believe that cherries may be an effective anti-inflammatory, along with helping support normal sleep, memory, arthritis, and may also help prevent cancer.

Cranberry – High in Vitamins C and K, cranberries are a good source of iodine and manganese. They also contain quinine, which helps purify the liver, prostate, kidneys, and bladder.

Dates – Along with being a great source of Vitamin B6, dates are high in minerals, including potassium, magnesium, copper, manganese, and iron. They also include important phytochemicals, like flavonoids, carotenoids, and phenolic acid. Researchers believe dates are good for brain health, inflammation, heart health, vision, and may have anti-cancer potential.

Grape – (red, black, concord, green) All grapes are good sources for Vitamin K, manganese, and potassium. Dark grapes, such as red grapes and concord grapes, are especially rich in flavonoids. Researchers believe that these flavonoids help reduce the amount of plaque in blood vessels.

Grapefruit – One of nature's best sources of Vitamin C, grapefruit also contains Vitamin A, potassium, thiamin, folate, and magnesium. It contains several anti-oxidants, including naringenin. Red varieties also contain lycopene, which is believed to support heart health and may have anti-cancer properties.

Honeydew Melon – Very high in Vitamin C, B6, thiamin, niacin, and folate, honeydew is also packed with the minerals, potassium and copper, thought to be good for radiant-looking skin.

Jujube – The Chinese date is high in Vitamin C and potassium. They are consumed in Asia to help decrease anxiety and improve sleep.

Kiwi – Kiwis are loaded with nutrients, including more Vitamin C than oranges, more potassium than bananas, plus Vitamin E, copper, magnesium, and phosphorous. Kiwi seeds contain high levels of omega-3 fatty acids. The green kiwi also contains chlorophyl. Researchers believe that kiwis support lung function and may have anti-cancer effects.

Lemon – Lemons are not only one of nature's best sources of Vitamin C, they are also high in folate and potassium. They contain the phytochemical limonene, thought to have anti-cancer properties.

Lime – Although they have distinctly different tastes, limes contain essentially the same nutrients as lemons, including Vitamin C, folate, and potassium.

Nectarine – Nectarines are a good source for Vitamins C, E, and B vitamins. The also provide potassium, and antioxidants like flavonoids, anthocyanins, and phenolic acids. Researchers believe that they enhance immunity, protect vision, and support healthy skin.

Orange – (mandarin, blood, juice) All varieties of orange are high in vitamin C, folate acid, and potassium. They also contain the antioxidants, hesperidin and limonoid. Researchers believe that oranges support immune function and help to reduce bad, LDL cholesterol.

Peach – The peach contains almost the same nutrients as the nectarine, including Vitamin C and A, niacin, potassium, and the antioxidants, lutein and lycopene.

Pear – Along with Vitamin C, pear is a good source of Vitamin E, riboflavin, potassium, and copper. Pear also contains pectin, which is a prebiotic that supports gastrointestinal health. Researchers believe that pear helps to lower bad, LDL cholesterol, supports brain health, and may protect against cancer.

Persimmon – An excellent source of the B Vitamins riboflavin, folate, and thiamin, persimmons are also high in Vitamins A, C, E, K, and the minerals potassium, copper, phosphorous, and manganese. They also contain a number of powerful antioxidants and are believed to support heart health.

Plum – Plums are rich in Vitamins C, A, and K. They also contain pectin, which supports gastrointestinal health. Plums also contain the phytochemicals chlorogenic acid and neochlorogenic acid, two powerful antioxidants which are believed to have anti-cancer effects.

Pomegranate – These delicious fruits are packed with nutrients, including Vitamins C and K, plus riboflavin, thiamin, and niacin. They also contain calcium and phosphorous. Researchers believe that pomegranates help to reduce plaque in blood vessels, in support of heart health. They also contain antioxidants, including tannins.

Pomelo – This big, sweet citrus is packed with Vitamins C, thiamin, and riboflavin. It also contains the minerals potassium and copper. Pomelos are rich in antioxidants and are believed to support heart health.

Raspberry – These beautiful berries are rich in Vitamins C and K, and contain the minerals manganese and magnesium. Raspberries contain high concentrations of ellagic acid, which is believed to boost immunity and have anti-cancer properties. Raspberries are also believed to support heart health.

Strawberry – The beloved strawberry is rich in Vitamin C and folate. They also contain potassium, sodium, and manganese. Strawberries contain antioxidants that are believed to support brain health.

Watermelon – The king of melons is rich in Vitamins A, C, B1, and B6, along with the minerals, potassium, magnesium, iodine and zinc. It also contains chlorophyl and lycopene, both powerful antioxidants. Watermelon is believed to support longevity and protect against certain types of cancer.

Vegetables:

Beet – This hardy root vegetable is a good source of Vitamins C, folate, and B6, plus the minerals, manganese, potassium, iron, calcium, and copper. It also contains antioxidants like betaine. Betaine is a substance found in the human body and some fruits and vegetables, that helps break down pathogens and harmful substances. Consumption of beet juice is associated with improved athletic performance, lower cholesterol, and liver health.

Bell Pepper – Bell peppers contain the Vitamins A, C, B6, K, E, and folate, along with potassium. They also contain a rich array of antioxidants, including capsanthin, violaxanthin, lutein, quercetin, and luteolin.

Broccoli – Rich in Vitamins C, A, and B1, broccoli also contains the minerals iron, calcium, sulfur, and potassium. It also contains two very potent phytochemicals, sulforaphane, and indoles. These two ingredients have been thoroughly researched for their anti-cancer properties. They are also believed to reduce arterial plaque, thus promoting heart health.

Burdock Root – Burdock contains the vitamins B6, folate, C, and the minerals manganese, potassium, phosphorous, calcium, and iron. It is also high in antioxidants, like quercetin, luteolin, and phenolic acids. Burdock has been used in traditional medicine systems for centuries for detox and cancer prevention.

Carrot – Along with Vitamin A (beta-carotene), carrot juice is also an excellent source for the B Complex vitamins, plus C, and K. It also contains the minerals calcium, sodium, phosphorous, and potassium. Carrot juice alkalizes blood, benefits vision, detoxes the liver and GI tract, and lowers cholesterol. It is also used for anti-anxiety.

Cauliflower – Cauliflower contains the Vitamins C, K, B6, folate, and pantothenic acid. It also has the minerals potassium, manganese, magnesium, and phosphorous. It also contains high concentrations of two antioxidants that are believed to slow the growth of cancer cells, glucosinolates, and isothiocyanates, as well and the antioxidants carotenoids and flavonoids.

Celery – These green stalks contain chlorophyl, along with Vitamins C, B1, B6, and folic acid. They also contain the minerals sodium and potassium. Celery also contains the phytochemical coumarin, which is believed to support heart health by helping to regulate blood pressure.

Chard – Chard is packed with nutrients, including the Vitamins A, C, K, E, B6, riboflavin, thiamin, and folic acid. It also is rich in the minerals iron, calcium, magnesium, phosphorous, potassium, copper, zinc, and manganese. Chard is believed to support bone and kidney health.

Chili Pepper – Chile peppers are rich in Vitamins C, A, B6, K, E, riboflavin, thiamin, and folic acid. It also contains the minerals potassium and magnesium. They also contain the powerful antioxidants, beta-cryptoxanthin, lutein, and zeaxanthin. Chiles help with symptoms of arthritis, and have been shown to reduce bad LDL cholesterol in support of heart health.

Cilantro – This tasty herb is rich in Vitamins A, C, E, K, and folic acid. It also contains the minerals potassium, calcium, iron, and magnesium. Cilantro is believed to support heart health by lowering cholesterol and by helping to regulate blood pressure. It is also used for anti-anxiety.

Collard Green – The garden contains few veggies that are as nutrient-rich as collard greens. Beside the generous amount of chlorophyl, collard greens contain the Vitamins A, C, B6, K, and folic acid, along with the minerals, calcium, magnesium, and sodium. They also contain the phytochemicals lutein and zeaxanthin, known to support healthy vision.

Cucumber – The reason that spas put little cucumber slices on your eyes is that cucumbers contain silicon, believed to be good for skin, hair, and nails. It's also good for connective tissue, like bones, tendons, and ligaments. Cucumbers also contain the Vitamins A, C, and K, along with the minerals phosphorous, manganese, magnesium, and potassium. Cucumbers contain sterols, which are thought to help reduce cholesterol.

Dandelion Green – These green leaves are more than lawn weeds. They contain a significant amount of Omega-3 and Omega-6 fatty acids. They also include the Vitamins A, C, E, and K, plus the minerals, calcium, iron, phosphorous, magnesium, potassium, and sodium.

Endive – Endive is loaded with Vitamins A, C, E, K, thiamin, riboflavin, and folic acid, along with the minerals, calcium, iron, magnesium, potassium, copper, manganese, and zinc. It also contains Omega-3 and Omega-6 fatty acids.

Fennel – Fennel contains phytoestrogens, which makes it a great addition to the diets of women who are pregnant, breastfeeding, or who are experiencing the symptoms associated with menopause. It contains the Vitamins C, niacin, and folic acid, along with the minerals, potassium, manganese, magnesium, and iron. It is associated with relieving cramps and digestive disorders.

Garlic – Garlic contains the phytochemical allicin, which researchers believe reduces the amount of plaque in blood vessels, lowers cholesterol, and helps regulate blood pressure. It is also used for detox and as an immune booster. It contains the Vitamins C and B6, along with the minerals, selenium, manganese, phosphorous, iron, copper, and potassium.

Ginger – Ginger contains phytochemicals known as gingerols, which researchers believe have strong anti-inflammatory properties, and is often consumed by arthritis sufferers. It contains a significant amount of Vitamin C, along with the minerals, copper, magnesium, and potassium.

Green Lettuce – Green lettuce varieties, like Romaine, contain carotenoids, which researchers believe inhibit certain types of cancers. Lettuce contains the Vitamins A, C, K, thiamin, folic acid, riboflavin, and B6, along with the minerals iron, potassium, manganese, calcium, copper, and magnesium. And let us not forget chlorophyll, nature's blood builder.

Green Onion – Green onions contain the vitamins A, B6, folic acid, C, and K, along with the minerals, calcium, manganese, and potassium. They also contain the phytochemical organosulfer, which researchers believe may have cancer-prevention properties.

Kale – Kale is packed with nutrients, including the Vitamins A, C, K, riboflavin, thiamin, and folic acid, along with the minerals, calcium, iron, manganese, phosphorous. potassium, copper, and magnesium. It also contains phytochemicals, such as chlorophyll, zeaxanthin, and a generous amount of lutein, which is good for the eyes. Kale has seven times more beta-carotene than broccoli.

Leek – Leeks contain the Vitamins A, C, K, and folic acid, with the minerals, manganese, magnesium, and iron. It also contains the phytochemicals quercetin and kaempferol, both believed to reduce the risk of developing various types of cancer, including ovarian cancer.

Radish – Radish juice is often consumed during a detox session. It contains the Vitamins C, folic acid, and riboflavin, with the minerals, potassium, calcium, manganese, and copper.

Rhubarb – Sometimes a vegetable, sometimes a fruit, rhubarb is loaded with nutrients including the Vitamins C, K, and folic acid, along with the minerals, calcium and potassium. Rhubarb contains several potent antioxidants, including tannins, and a higher polyphenol content than kale. It also contains anthocyanins, which are responsible for its red color, and thought to have numerous health benefits.

Shallot – Shallots have a more robust nutritional profile than their onion cousins, and contain a significant amount of allicin, which researchers believe lowers cholesterol. They also contain the Vitamins A, C, folic acid, niacin, pantothenic acid, thiamin, and riboflavin, along with the minerals, sodium, potassium, calcium, iron, copper, magnesium, manganese, selenium, zinc, and phosphorous.

Spinach – Spinach contains powerful antioxidants, such as glutathione, referred to by some researchers as 'nature's master antioxidant'. It is a biological molecule found in cells which protects DNA, while it boosts immune response and reduces chronic inflammation. Spinach contains the Vitamins A, C, E, and folic acid, along with the minerals, calcium and potassium. Spinach also contains other important phytochemicals, such as chlorophyll, lutein, choline, and alpha lipoic acid.

Squash – The many varieties of squash, all have a similar nutritional profile. Zucchini, for example, contains the Vitamins A, C, E, B6, folic acid, and K, along with the minerals, potassium, calcium, iron, magnesium, and manganese. It also contains Omega-3 and Omega-6 fatty acids.

Sprout Grass – Wheat grass and barley grass are two of the most nutrient rich food sources there are. Vitamins in sprout grass include C, K, E, thiamin, riboflavin, B12, niacin, pantothenic acid, folic acid, and biotin. Minerals contained in sprout grass include calcium, phosphorous, potassium, magnesium, iron, manganese, selenium, sodium, iodine, zinc, copper, and cobalt. Sprout grass is also rich in amino acids.

Tomatillos – Tomatillos are packed with generous amounts of Vitamins, including A, C, E, K, thiamin, niacin, and folic acid, along with the minerals, calcium, copper, iron, magnesium, manganese, phosphorous, selenium, and zinc. It also contains the phytonutrients, lutein-zeaxanthin, carotene, and lycopene.

Tomato – Tomato juice gets its red color from lycopene, one of the most potent antioxidants in all of nature. It is also rich in Vitamins C, and the minerals, sodium, potassium, calcium, magnesium, and sulfur.

Turnip – Researchers believe that turnips help to regulate blood pressure and support gastrointestinal health. Turnips contain the Vitamins C, K, and folic acid, along with the minerals, calcium, iron, magnesium, phosphorous, sodium, and zinc.